UNDERSTANDING HIGH BLOOD PRESSURE

Understanding, Managing, and Overcoming It for the Best Possible Health and Wellness in 2023–2024

TEMMY JOHN

Table of Contents:

1. introduction

High blood pressure, often referred to as hypertension, is a silent yet pervasive threat that affects millions of individuals worldwide. While it may not manifest obvious symptoms in its early stages, its long-term consequences can be severe, leading to cardiovascular disease, stroke, and other life-threatening complications. In this comprehensive introduction, we delve into the intricacies of high blood pressure, exploring its causes, risk factors, symptoms, and management strategies.

The Basics of Blood Pressure

The force that blood exerts on the artery walls while it circulates throughout the body is known as blood pressure. It consists of two components: systolic pressure, which measures the force when the heart contracts, and diastolic pressure, which measures the force when the heart relaxes between beats. Blood pressure readings are typically expressed as systolic over diastolic (e.g., 120/80 mmHg), with normal values falling below 120/80 mmHg.

Understanding Hypertension

Hypertension occurs when blood pressure remains consistently elevated over time, placing increased strain on the heart and blood vessels. While normal blood pressure is vital for delivering oxygen and nutrients to the body's tissues, persistent hypertension can damage the arteries, heart, brain, kidneys, and other organs, setting the stage for a variety of serious health problems.

Risk Factors and Causes

Numerous factors contribute to the development of high blood pressure, including genetics, age, lifestyle choices, and underlying health conditions. Family history, advancing age, and certain medical conditions such as diabetes, kidney disease, and sleep apnea can elevate the risk of hypertension. Additionally, lifestyle factors such as poor diet, lack of physical activity, excess weight, tobacco use, and high alcohol consumption are significant contributors to elevated blood pressure.

Symptoms and Complications

One of the most insidious aspects of high blood pressure is its often asymptomatic nature, earning it the moniker of "the silent killer." Many individuals with hypertension may not experience any noticeable symptoms until complications arise. However, as blood pressure climbs to dangerously high levels, symptoms such as headaches, dizziness, shortness of breath, blurred vision, and chest pain may manifest. If left untreated, hypertension can lead to severe complications, including heart attack, stroke, heart failure, kidney disease, and vision loss.

Diagnosis and Monitoring

It is crucial to regularly check blood pressure in order to diagnose and treat hypertension. Blood pressure readings can be obtained using a sphygmomanometer, a device that measures pressure in the arteries, or through automated blood pressure monitors. Diagnosis typically requires multiple readings taken over time to establish a pattern of elevated blood pressure. Additionally, healthcare providers may recommend further tests to assess organ damage and identify underlying conditions contributing to hypertension.

Management and Treatment

The management of high blood pressure often involves a multifaceted approach aimed at reducing blood pressure levels and minimizing the risk of complications. Lifestyle modifications such as adopting a healthy diet rich in fruits, vegetables, whole grains, and lean proteins, maintaining a healthy weight, engaging in regular physical activity, limiting sodium intake, moderating alcohol consumption, and quitting smoking are crucial components of hypertension management.

In conclusion, high blood pressure represents a significant public health concern with far-reaching implications for global health. While it may initially go unnoticed, the long-term consequences of untreated hypertension can be devastating. By understanding the basics of blood pressure, recognizing risk factors, and implementing effective management strategies, individuals can take proactive steps to safeguard their cardiovascular health and reduce the burden of this silent yet formidable adversary.

2. What is High Blood Pressure?

High blood pressure, also known as hypertension, is a medical condition characterized by elevated pressure in the arteries as the heart pumps blood throughout the body. The two numbers that represent blood pressure are the diastolic pressure (the bottom number), which indicates the pressure in the arteries between heartbeats, and the systolic pressure (the top number), which indicates the pressure in the arteries during a heartbeat.

Normal blood pressure is typically around 120/80 mm Hg (millimeters of mercury). However, when blood pressure consistently exceeds 130/80 mm Hg, it is considered elevated and may indicate the presence of hypertension. High blood pressure puts added strain on the heart and blood vessels, increasing the risk of various health complications, including heart disease, stroke, kidney damage, and vision problems.

Primary hypertension, or essential hypertension, and secondary hypertension are the two main forms of high blood pressure. The bulk of cases, known as primary hypertension, occur gradually over time and lack a clear underlying reason.` Secondary hypertension is usually caused by an underlying condition, such as kidney disease, hormonal disorders, or certain medications.

Monitoring blood pressure regularly, adopting a healthy lifestyle, maintaining a balanced diet, staying physically active, managing stress, and following medical advice are crucial for controlling high blood pressure. By understanding what high blood pressure is and how it impacts overall health, individuals can take steps to manage the condition effectively and reduce the risk of associated complications.

3. Causes and Risk Factors

I'm glad to provide you with detailed information on the causes and risk factors associated with high blood pressure.

High blood pressure, or hypertension, can be influenced by a variety of factors, including both controllable lifestyle choices and uncontrollable genetic predispositions. Understanding the causes and risk factors of hypertension is essential for effectively managing and potentially preventing this common health condition.

Causes of High Blood Pressure:

1. Genetics: Family history plays a significant role in the development of high blood pressure. People who have a family history of hypertension are at an increased risk of developing the illness themselves.

2. Age: Blood pressure tends to rise with age due to changes in artery stiffness and the overall function of the cardiovascular system.

3. Lifestyle factors: Unhealthy lifestyle choices, including a diet high in sodium, unhealthy fats, and refined sugars, as well as lack of physical activity, can contribute to the development of high blood pressure.

4. Obesity: Excess weight, especially around the abdomen, puts stress on the heart and circulatory system, leading to an increased risk of hypertension.

5. Smoking: Tobacco use and exposure to secondhand smoke can raise blood pressure and damage blood vessels, increasing the risk of hypertension.

6. Stress: Chronic stress and high levels of cortisol (the stress hormone) can lead to elevated blood pressure over time.

7. Chronic conditions: Certain medical conditions, such as kidney disease, thyroid disorders, an
d sleep apnea, can contribute to hypertension.

Risk Factors for High Blood Pressure:

1. Age: The risk of developing high blood pressure increases with age, with adults over 65 being at higher risk.

2. Gender: Men have a higher risk of developing hypertension at a younger age, while women are more at risk after menopause.

3. Ethnicity: Some ethnic groups, such as African Americans, are at a higher risk of developing high blood pressure.

4. Family history: Individuals with a family history of hypertension are more likely to develop the condition themselves.

5. Sedentary lifestyle: Lack of regular physical activity can contribute to weight gain and high blood pressure.

6. Unhealthy diet: Diets high in sodium, saturated fats, and added sugars can increase the risk of hypertension.

7. Alcohol consumption: Excessive alcohol consumption can raise blood pressure and contribute to hypertension.

8. Chronic stress: Prolonged stress and anxiety can elevate blood pressure levels over time.

Understanding the causes and risk factors of high blood pressure is crucial for taking proactive steps to manage and reduce the risk of developing this condition. By addressing lifestyle factors, making healthy choices, and seeking appropriate medical care, individuals can work towards maintaining optimal blood pressure levels and overall cardiovascular health.

4. Symptoms and Signs of High Blood Pressure

High blood pressure, also known as hypertension, is often referred to as a "silent killer" because it typically does not cause noticeable symptoms until it reaches a severe stage. However, in some cases, individuals may experience subtle signs that could indicate high blood pressure and prompt further investigation. Understanding the symptoms and signs of high blood pressure is essential for early detection and effective management of this common health condition.

Symptoms of High Blood Pressure:

1. Headaches: Persistent headaches, especially at the back of the head, can be a symptom of high blood pressure. The headaches may be more severe in the morning.

2. Dizziness: Feeling lightheaded, dizzy, or experiencing vertigo can sometimes occur as a result of elevated blood pressure levels.

3. Shortness of breath: Difficulty breathing or shortness of breath, particularly with exertion or physical activity, can be a sign of underlying hypertension.

4. Chest pain: Chest pain or tightness may occur in individuals with high blood pressure, especially during periods of increased stress or physical strain.

5. Vision changes: Blurred vision, eye redness, or vision problems can sometimes be associated with high

blood pressure complications affecting the eyes.
6. Fatigue: Persistent fatigue, weakness, or feelings of exhaustion may be related to the strain that high blood pressure puts on the cardiovascular system.
7. Nosebleeds: Although less prevalent, frequent or inexplicable nosebleeds may occasionally be associated with problems with hypertension.
 Signs of High Blood Pressure:
1. Elevated blood pressure readings: The most reliable way to diagnose high blood pressure is through regular blood pressure measurements. Elevated readings consistently above 130/80 mm Hg indicate hypertension.
2. Uncontrolled stress: Chronic stress, anxiety, and tension can contribute to elevated blood pressure levels over time.
3. Increased heart rate: A rapid or irregular heart rate, also known as palpitations, can be a sign of elevated blood pressure and cardiovascular strain.
4. Flushing or redness: Redness or flushing of the face, particularly during periods of stress or physical activity, can indicate elevated blood pressure.
5. Swelling: Swelling in the legs, hands, or other parts of the body can occur as a result of hypertension-related complications.
It is important to note that high blood pressure is often asymptomatic or presents with non-specific symptoms, making regular blood pressure monitoring crucial for early detection and management. Maintaining a

healthy lifestyle, including a balanced diet, regular physical activity, stress management, and routine medical check-ups, can help prevent and control high blood pressure effectively. Prompt medical attention should be sought if any concerning symptoms or signs are experienced to prevent potential complications associated with hypertension.

5. Complications Associated with High Blood Pressure

High blood pressure, or hypertension, is a serious medical condition that, if left uncontrolled, can lead to a variety of complications affecting various organs and systems in the body. Understanding the potential complications associated with high blood pressure is crucial for motivating individuals to prioritize blood pressure management and adopt healthy lifestyle choices to reduce their risk.
 Complications of High Blood Pressure:
1. Heart Disease: One of the most significant complications of high blood pressure is heart disease. Elevated blood pressure puts strain on the heart, increasing the risk of coronary artery disease, heart attacks, and heart failure.
2. Stroke: Hypertension is a leading risk factor for stroke, a sudden interruption of blood flow to the brain. High blood pressure can cause blood vessels in the brain to weaken and rupture, leading to a stroke.

3. Kidney Damage: Chronic high blood pressure can damage the blood vessels in the kidneys, reducing their ability to function properly. This can lead to kidney disease or even kidney failure.

4. Vision Problems: Hypertension can affect the blood vessels in the eyes, leading to vision problems such as retinopathy, vision loss, or other eye-related complications.

5. Peripheral Artery Disease: High blood pressure can cause a narrowing of the arteries in the legs, arms, stomach, and head, leading to peripheral artery disease. This condition can result in reduced blood flow to these areas and may cause pain, numbness, or other symptoms.

6. Aneurysm: Chronic high blood pressure can weaken the walls of blood vessels, increasing the risk of aneurysms - bulges or balloon-like deformities in the blood vessels. A ruptured aneurysm can be life-threatening.

7. Cognitive Decline: Hypertension has been linked to an increased risk of cognitive decline and dementia, including Alzheimer's disease, due to reduced blood flow to the brain.

8. Metabolic Syndrome: High blood pressure is a key component of metabolic syndrome, a cluster of conditions that includes obesity, high blood sugar, and abnormal cholesterol levels.Type 2 diabetes, heart disease, and stroke are all made more likely by this syndrome.

9. Pregnancy Complications: High blood pressure during pregnancy, known as gestational hypertension or

preeclampsia, can lead to serious complications for both the mother and the baby, including preterm birth and low birth weight.

10. Sleep Apnea: Hypertension is often associated with sleep apnea, a sleep disorder characterized by pauses in breathing during sleep. Sleep apnea can contribute to high blood pressure and vice versa.

By understanding the potential complications of high blood pressure, individuals can be more motivated to engage in preventive measures, such as maintaining a healthy lifestyle, monitoring blood pressure regularly, and seeking medical treatment when necessary. Managing high blood pressure effectively can significantly reduce the risk of developing these serious complications and improve overall health outcomes.

6. Diagnosis of High Blood Pressure

Diagnosing high blood pressure, also known as hypertension, is a critical step in managing and controlling this common health condition. Regular blood pressure monitoring and proper diagnostic procedures are essential for identifying elevated blood pressure levels and initiating appropriate interventions to prevent complications. Here is an overview of the diagnosis of high blood pressure:

Diagnostic Methods for High Blood Pressure:

1. Blood Pressure Measurement:
   - Blood pressure is measured using a device called a sphygmomanometer,

which provides readings in millimeters of mercury (mm Hg).The two figures in a blood pressure reading are the diastolic pressure, which is the bottom number, and the systolic pressure, which is the top number. For instance, 120/80 mm Hg is regarded as normal.

- Blood pressure can be measured using manual or electronic devices. Systolic and diastolic pressures are recorded to determine overall blood pressure levels.

2. Classification of Blood Pressure:

- Blood pressure is classified into different categories based on the readings obtained during measurement. Normal blood pressure, increased blood pressure, stage 1 hypertension, and stage 2 hypertension are among these classifications.

3. Repeat Measurements:

- To confirm a diagnosis of high blood pressure, healthcare providers may conduct multiple blood pressure measurements on separate occasions. This helps to account for factors like white coat hypertension (elevated blood pressure in a clinical setting) and ensure an accurate diagnosis.

4. Home Blood Pressure Monitoring:

- Home blood pressure monitoring is recommended for individuals with suspected high blood pressure or those already diagnosed with the condition. Regular monitoring at home can provide valuable data for healthcare providers and help individuals track their blood pressure levels effectively.

5. Ambulatory Blood Pressure
Monitoring:
   - In some cases, ambulatory blood
pressure monitoring may be used to
assess blood pressure levels over a
24-hour period. This method provides
a more comprehensive evaluation of
blood pressure throughout the day
and night.
6. Additional Testing:
   - Healthcare providers may
recommend additional tests to assess
the impact of high blood pressure on
target organs, such as the heart,
kidneys, and blood vessels. Tests may
include blood tests, electrocardiogram
(ECG), echocardiogram, and
ultrasound scans.
7. Diagnostic Criteria:
   - Healthcare professionals use
diagnostic criteria from organizations
such as the American Heart
Association (AHA) and the American
College of Cardiology (ACC) to
determine appropriate thresholds for
diagnosing high blood pressure.
Diagnosing high blood pressure in a
timely manner is crucial for initiating
appropriate treatment and lifestyle
modifications to manage the condition
effectively. Regular monitoring,
accurate measurement techniques,
and collaboration with healthcare
providers are key components of the
diagnostic process for high blood
pressure.

7. Treatment Options for High Blood Pressure

Treating high blood pressure, or
hypertension, is crucial for reducing

the risk of complications and improving overall health outcomes. A combination of lifestyle changes, medications, and sometimes alternative therapies is typically used to manage high blood pressure effectively. Here are some common treatment options for high blood pressure:

Treatment Options for High Blood Pressure:

7.1 Lifestyle Changes

- Dietary Modifications: Adopting a heart-healthy diet rich in fruits, vegetables, whole grains, lean proteins, and low-fat dairy can help lower blood pressure. Limiting sodium intake, avoiding processed foods, and reducing alcohol consumption are also beneficial.

- Regular Exercise: Engaging in regular physical activity, such as brisk walking, cycling, swimming, or strength training, can help lower blood pressure. Try to get in at least 150 minutes a week of moderate-to-intense activity.

- Weight Management: Maintaining a healthy weight through a balanced diet and consistent physical activity can reduce the strain on the heart and blood vessels, leading to lower blood pressure levels.

- Stress Management: Techniques such as deep breathing, meditation, yoga, and mindfulness can help reduce stress levels, which in turn may lower blood pressure.

7.2 Medications:

- Diuretics: By assisting the body in getting rid of extra salt and water, these drugs lower blood pressure and volume of blood.

- Beta-Blockers: These medications reduce nerve signals to the heart and blood vessels, lowering heart rate and blood pressure.

- Calcium Channel Blockers: These medications relax blood vessels and reduce the heart's workload, leading to decreased blood pressure.

- ACE Inhibitors and ARBs: These medications relax blood vessels by blocking the effects of certain hormones, helping blood vessels dilate and lower blood pressure.

- Combination Therapies: In some cases, a combination of medications may be prescribed to effectively control high blood pressure.

7.3 Alternative Therapies:
- Mind-Body Techniques: Practices such as yoga, tai chi, biofeedback, and meditation may help reduce stress and lower blood pressure.

- Herbal Supplements: Certain herbal supplements like garlic extract, hawthorn, and fish oil may have modest blood-pressure-lowering effects, but it's important to consult with a healthcare provider before using them.

7.4 Regular Monitoring:
- Monitoring blood pressure regularly at home and during medical check-ups is vital for tracking the

effectiveness of treatment and adjusting interventions as needed.

7.5 Medical Supervision:

- Working closely with healthcare providers, including doctors, nurses, and pharmacists, is essential for optimizing high blood pressure treatment and managing potential side effects of medications.

By incorporating a combination of lifestyle modifications, medications, and alternative therapies, individuals can effectively manage high blood pressure and reduce the risk of associated complications. It's important to follow the treatment plan recommended by healthcare providers

8. Prevention and Management Strategies

Preventing and managing high blood pressure, or hypertension, is essential for reducing the risk of cardiovascular complications and promoting overall health. By adopting healthy lifestyle habits, monitoring blood pressure regularly, and seeking medical guidance when necessary, individuals can take proactive steps to prevent and manage high blood pressure effectively. Here are key prevention and management strategies for high blood pressure:

Prevention Strategies:

1. Healthy Diet:

- Keep a healthy, well-balanced diet full of whole grains, fruits, vegetables, lean meats, low-fat dairy products, and other nutrients.

- Reduce sodium intake by avoiding processed foods, salty snacks, and excessive use of table salt.

- Limit consumption of sugary beverages, saturated fats, and foods high in cholesterol.

2. Regular Physical Activity:

- Engage in moderate-intensity exercise for at least 150 minutes per week, or vigorous-intensity exercise for 75 minutes per week.

- Include activities like brisk walking, jogging, swimming, cycling, or aerobics to promote cardiovascular health.

3. Weight Management:

- Eat a balanced diet and get regular exercise to help you maintain a healthy weight.

- Aim for a body mass index (BMI) within the healthy range to reduce the risk of hypertension.

4. Stress Management:

- Practice stress-reduction techniques such as deep breathing, meditation, yoga, or mindfulness to lower stress levels and promote relaxation.

- To enhance mental health, give self-care, hobbies, and social contacts top priority.

5. Limit Alcohol and Tobacco Use:

- Keep alcohol intake in moderation because too much of it can elevate blood pressure.

- Quit smoking and avoid exposure to secondhand smoke to reduce the risk of hypertension and cardiovascular disease.

Management Strategies:

1. Regular Blood Pressure Monitoring:

- Monitor blood pressure regularly at home using a reliable blood pressure monitor and keep track of readings over time.
- Maintain a blood pressure log and share the information with healthcare providers during check-ups.

2. Medication Adherence:
- Adhere to doctor's orders when using prescription drugs, and never miss a dosage.
- Report any side effects or concerns about medications to healthcare professionals for timely adjustments.

3. Healthy Lifestyle Practices:
- Continue following a heart-healthy diet, engaging in regular physical activity, and managing stress effectively.
- Incorporate relaxation techniques, hobbies, and social support to maintain overall well-being.

4. Regular Medical Check-ups:
- Attend routine medical check-ups to monitor blood pressure, assess overall health, and receive guidance on managing hypertension.
- Stay informed about blood pressure readings, test results, and treatment recommendations from healthcare providers.

By integrating these prevention and management strategies into daily routines, individuals can empower themselves to prevent high blood pressure, maintain optimal blood pressure levels, and reduce the risk of associated health complications. Consistent effort and commitment to a healthy lifestyle are key to managing high blood pressure effectively and promoting

8.1 Dietary Recommendations

Diet plays a crucial role in managing high blood pressure and promoting cardiovascular health. Making dietary changes to include foods that support healthy blood pressure levels can significantly impact overall well-being. Here are some dietary recommendations for preventing and managing high blood pressure:

Dietary Recommendations for High Blood Pressure:

1. Limit Sodium Intake:
   - Reduce the consumption of high-sodium foods such as processed meats, canned soups, salty snacks, and fast food.
   - Opt for low-sodium alternatives and choose fresh, whole foods to control sodium intake.

2. Increase Potassium-Rich Foods:
   - Include potassium-rich foods in your diet, such as bananas, avocados, sweet potatoes, spinach, and tomatoes.
   - Potassium helps counterbalance the effects of sodium and supports healthy blood pressure levels.

3. Eat Magnesium-Rich Foods:
   - Magnesium-rich foods like leafy greens, nuts, seeds, whole grains, and legumes can help regulate blood pressure and promote heart health.
   - Incorporate these foods into your diet to support overall cardiovascular function.

4. Focus on Fruits and Vegetables:

- Try to have half of your plate composed of a range of vibrant, high-nutrient fruits and veggies.
   - These nutrient-dense foods help lower blood pressure and reduce the risk of heart disease.
5. Choose Lean Proteins:
   - Opt for lean protein sources such as poultry, fish, tofu, legumes, and low-fat dairy to support muscle health and maintain a balanced diet.
   - Limit red meat consumption and opt for healthier protein alternatives.
6. Whole Grains and Fiber:
   - Incorporate whole grains like oats, quinoa, brown rice, and whole wheat bread to increase fiber intake and support heart health.
   - Diets high in fiber promote better digestive health and reduce cholesterol.
7. Healthy Fats:
   - Include sources of healthy fats like olive oil, avocado, nuts, seeds, and fatty fish such as salmon and mackerel.
   - These unsaturated fats can help reduce inflammation, lower cholesterol, and support overall heart function.
8. Limit Saturated and Trans Fats:
   - Minimize intake of saturated fats found in red meat, butter, and full-fat dairy products, as well as trans fats in processed foods and baked goods.
   - Choose healthier fat sources to reduce the risk of cardiovascular disease.
9. Stay Hydrated:
   - Drink an adequate amount of water throughout the day to stay hydrated

and support optimal blood pressure levels.

- Limit sugary beverages, caffeinated drinks, and alcohol consumption to maintain hydration and overall health.

By following these dietary recommendations and making informed choices about food selection, individuals can improve their blood pressure levels, support cardiovascular health, and reduce the risk of hypertension-related complications. Incorporating a variety of nutrient-dense foods into daily meals can contribute to long

8.2 Exercise Guidelines

Engaging in regular physical activity is a key component of managing high blood pressure and promoting overall cardiovascular health. Exercise can help lower blood pressure, improve heart function, increase cardiovascular fitness, and contribute to overall well-being. Here are some exercise guidelines for individuals with high blood pressure:

Exercise Guidelines for High Blood Pressure:

1. Aerobic Exercise:

- Aim for 150 minutes or more each week of moderate-to-intense aerobic activity, such as dance, swimming, cycling, or brisk walking.

- Alternatively, target 75 minutes of vigorous-intensity aerobic activity weekly for optimal cardiovascular benefits.

2. Strength Training:

- Include strength training exercises at least two days per week to build muscle strength, improve metabolism, and support overall health.
   - Use free weights, resistance bands, machines, or bodyweight exercises to target major muscle groups.
3. Flexibility and Balance Exercises:
   - Incorporate stretching exercises to improve flexibility and mobility, reducing the risk of injury and supporting joint health.
   - Practice balance exercises to enhance stability, coordination, and posture.
4. Gradual Progression:
- Start slowly and gradually increase the duration, intensity, and frequency of exercise sessions to avoid overexertion and allow the body to adapt.
   - Listen to your body, and adjust your exercise routine based on your fitness level and comfort.
5. Warm-Up and Cool Down:
   - Always begin with a gentle warm-up, such as walking or light stretching, to prepare the body for exercise and prevent injury.
   - Conclude each exercise session with a proper cool-down, including stretching and relaxation techniques to help the body recover.
6. Consistency and Variety:
   - Strive for consistent exercise habits by scheduling regular workouts throughout the week and maintaining a balanced routine.
   - Include a variety of exercises to target different muscle groups, prevent

boredom, and maximize health benefits.

7. Monitoring Intensity:

   - Use the Borg Rating of Perceived Exertion (RPE) scale or a heart rate monitor to guide exercise intensity and ensure you are working at a safe and effective level.

   - Aim for a moderate level of intensity (corresponding to a perceived exertion of around 5-6 on a scale of 0-10) for most aerobic activities.

8. Consult with Healthcare Providers:

   - Before starting an exercise program, consult with your healthcare provider, especially if you have existing health conditions or concerns about exercising with high blood pressure.

   - Discuss personalized exercise recommendations and modifications based on your individual health status. By following these exercise guidelines and incorporating physical activity into your daily routine, you can help manage high blood pressure, improve cardiovascular fitness, and enhance overall health and well-being. Regular exercise, combined with a balanced diet and other healthy lifestyle choices, plays a vital role in supporting optimal blood pressure levels and reducing the risk of hypertension-related complications.

8.3 Stress Management Techniques

Effectively managing stress is crucial for overall well-being, including the management of high blood pressure.

Chronic stress can contribute to elevated blood pressure levels and increase the risk of cardiovascular issues. Implementing stress management techniques can help individuals reduce stress, promote relaxation, and support optimal cardiovascular health. Here are some stress management techniques that can be beneficial for individuals with high blood pressure:
 Stress Management Techniques for High Blood Pressure:
1. Mindfulness Meditation:
   - Practice mindfulness meditation to focus on the present moment, cultivate awareness, and promote relaxation.
   - Engage in deep breathing exercises, body scans, or guided meditation to reduce stress and calm the mind.
2. Yoga and Tai Chi:
   - Participate in yoga or tai chi classes to improve flexibility, reduce tension, and enhance relaxation.
   - These mind-body practices combine physical movements with breath awareness to promote mental and physical well-being.
3. Progressive Muscle Relaxation:
 Tensing and then relaxing each muscle group in the body is a technique known as progressive muscle relaxation.
   - This technique can help release physical tension, reduce stress, and induce a state of relaxation.
4. Physical Activity:
   - Engage in regular physical exercise, such as walking, jogging,

cycling, or swimming, to release endorphins and reduce stress levels.
   - Exercise can boost mood, improve sleep quality, and provide a natural outlet for stress relief.
5. Healthy Lifestyle Habits:
   - Maintain a balanced diet, get an adequate amount of sleep, and stay hydrated to promote overall well-being and reduce the impact of stress.
   - Avoid excessive caffeine and alcohol consumption, as they can worsen stress and anxiety.
6. Journaling and Expressive Writing:
   - Keep a journal to write down thoughts, feelings, and experiences as a way to process emotions and gain insight into sources of stress.
   - Reflect on positive experiences, express gratitude, and set achievable goals to encourage a positive mindset.
7. Social Support:
   - Seek support from friends, family members, or mental health professionals to share concerns, receive guidance, and build a supportive network.
   - Connecting with others can help alleviate feelings of isolation, reduce stress, and foster a sense of belonging.
8. Time Management and Prioritization:
   - Practice effective time management techniques, such as prioritizing tasks, setting boundaries, and delegating responsibilities.
   - Break tasks into manageable steps, set realistic goals, and focus on one task at a time to reduce overwhelm and stress.

By incorporating these stress management techniques into daily routines, individuals can reduce stress, improve emotional well-being, and support optimal blood pressure levels. Managing stress effectively is a key component of maintaining overall health and promoting cardiovascular wellness.

9. Monitoring High Blood Pressure

Monitoring high blood pressure on a regular basis is essential for individuals with hypertension to track their blood pressure levels, assess the effectiveness of treatment, and identify any changes or fluctuations that may require adjustments in management. Consistent monitoring allows individuals to take proactive steps in managing their condition and reducing the risk of associated complications. Here are some important aspects of monitoring high blood pressure:
 Monitoring High Blood Pressure:
1. Frequency of Monitoring:
   - Individuals with high blood pressure should monitor their blood pressure as recommended by their healthcare provider. This may involve daily monitoring at home or periodic checks during medical visits.
2. Home Blood Pressure Monitoring:
   - Home blood pressure monitoring is a valuable tool for tracking blood pressure levels between medical appointments. It allows individuals to observe patterns, identify changes, and provide accurate data to healthcare providers.

3. Choosing a Reliable Blood Pressure Monitor:
   - Use a validated and properly calibrated blood pressure monitor to ensure accurate readings. Automatic digital monitors are user-friendly and offer consistent results.

4. Tracking Blood Pressure Readings:
   - Record blood pressure readings in a logbook or a digital app to monitor trends over time. Include dates, time of day, readings, and any relevant information such as activities, medications, or symptoms.

5. Healthy Environment for Monitoring:
   - Create a calm and quiet environment for blood pressure measurements. Sit quietly for a few minutes before taking readings and avoid caffeine, tobacco, or exercise beforehand.

6. Consistent Measurement Technique:
   - Follow the recommended measurement technique, such as placing the cuff at heart level, keeping legs uncrossed, and ensuring a proper fit for accurate readings.

7. Understanding Blood Pressure Readings:
   - Learn about blood pressure readings, including the significance of systolic and diastolic numbers, target ranges for different categories of blood pressure, and the implications of high or low readings.

8. Communication with Healthcare Providers:
   - Share blood pressure logs and any concerns with healthcare providers during check-ups or consultations.

Discuss any significant changes in readings, symptoms, or lifestyle factors impacting blood pressure.
9. Lifestyle Modifications Based on Readings:
   - Use blood pressure data to make informed decisions about medication adherence, dietary choices, physical activity, stress management, or other lifestyle modifications that may impact blood pressure levels.
10. Regular Medical Check-ups:
   - Regularly visit healthcare providers for comprehensive evaluations, blood pressure assessments, medication reviews, and personalized guidance on managing high blood pressure effectively.
By actively monitoring blood pressure levels, maintaining accurate records, and collaborating with healthcare providers, individuals with high blood pressure can stay informed about their health status, track progress in managing the condition, and make informed decisions to promote cardiovascular wellness. Monitoring high blood pressure is a proactive step towards maintaining optimal blood pressure levels and reducing the risk of complications associated with hypertension.

9.1 Home Blood Pressure Monitoring

Home blood pressure monitoring is a valuable tool for individuals with hypertension to track their blood pressure levels in the comfort of their own environment. Regular monitoring at home provides insights into blood pressure trends, helps in assessing the effectiveness of treatment strategies, and enables proactive management of high blood pressure. Here are some key aspects of home blood pressure monitoring:

Home Blood Pressure Monitoring:

1. Choosing the Right Blood Pressure Monitor:

   - Select a validated and properly calibrated blood pressure monitor that meets quality standards. Automatic digital monitors are commonly recommended for ease of use and accuracy.

2. Proper Technique:

   - Sit in a chair with your feet flat on the ground, your back supported, and your arm at heart level to ensure proper posture. Ensure a proper fit of the cuff on the upper arm for accurate readings.

3. Consistent Timing:

   - Monitor blood pressure at the same time each day, preferably in the morning and evening, or as advised by healthcare providers. Avoid measuring right after meals, caffeine consumption, or physical activity.

4. Relaxation and Rest:

   - Sit quietly for a few minutes before taking measurements to allow your body to relax. Refrain from talking or moving during the reading to obtain accurate results.

5. Multiple Readings:

   - Take two to three measurements, with a brief rest in between, and record the average reading. This helps account for variations and provides a more reliable representation of blood pressure.

6. Record Keeping:
   - Maintain a logbook or use a digital app to record blood pressure readings, including date, time, systolic and diastolic numbers, pulse rate, and any relevant notes on activities or symptoms.
7. Monitoring Trends:
   - Track trends in blood pressure levels over time to identify patterns, changes, or fluctuations. Note any factors influencing variations, such as stress, medication adherence, or lifestyle habits.
8. Communication with Healthcare Providers:
   - Share home blood pressure logs with healthcare providers during appointments or consultations. Discuss any concerns, notable readings, or changes in blood pressure patterns for personalized guidance.
9. Regular Reviews:
   - Review blood pressure monitoring data with healthcare providers to assess progress, adjust treatment plans if necessary, and receive recommendations on managing high blood pressure effectively.
10. Effective Use of Data:
   - Use home blood pressure monitoring data to make informed decisions about lifestyle modifications, medication adherence, stress management, and other factors impacting blood pressure control.
By embracing home blood pressure monitoring as part of a proactive approach to managing hypertension, individuals can empower themselves to monitor their health, engage in self-

care practices, and work collaboratively with healthcare providers towards achieving optimal blood pressure levels and overall cardiovascular wellness. The consistent and accurate monitoring of blood pressure at home contributes to better management of hypertension and reduces the risk of complications associated with high blood pressure.

9.2 Regular Check-ups

Regular check-ups are essential for individuals with high blood pressure to receive comprehensive evaluations, monitor blood pressure levels, assess overall health status, and collaborate with healthcare providers in managing hypertension effectively. These routine medical appointments play a vital role in preventing complications, optimizing treatment strategies, and promoting cardiovascular wellness. Here are key aspects of regular check-ups for individuals with high blood pressure:
Regular Check-ups for High Blood Pressure:
1. Scheduled Appointments:
   - Attend regular check-ups as recommended by healthcare providers to monitor blood pressure, assess cardiovascular health, and receive guidance on managing hypertension.
2. Blood Pressure Measurement:
   - Have blood pressure checked at each visit to monitor trends, evaluate control of hypertension, and make adjustments to treatment plans if necessary.
3. Medication Review:

- Review current medications, dosages, and potential side effects with healthcare providers to ensure optimal management of high blood pressure and address any concerns.

4. Lifestyle Assessment:

- Discuss lifestyle habits, including diet, exercise, stress management, alcohol consumption, and smoking, to identify areas for improvement and promote heart-healthy behaviors.

5. Symptom Evaluation:

- Report any symptoms or concerns related to high blood pressure, such as headaches, dizziness, chest pain, or changes in vision, for timely evaluation and intervention.

6. Risk Factor Assessment:

- Assess risk factors contributing to hypertension, such as family history, obesity, sedentary lifestyle, high sodium intake, and stress levels, to develop targeted interventions.

7. Comprehensive Testing:

- Undergo comprehensive evaluations, including blood tests, electrocardiograms, echocardiograms, and other diagnostic tests, to assess cardiovascular health and screen for potential complications.

8. Education and Counseling:

- Receive education on hypertension management, lifestyle modifications, medication adherence, and self-care practices to empower informed decision-making and promote long-term wellness.

9. Goal Setting:

- Collaborate with healthcare providers to establish realistic goals for blood pressure control, weight management, physical activity, dietary

changes, and stress reduction to achieve optimal health outcomes.
10. Follow-up Plans:
   - Establish follow-up plans and schedule future appointments to monitor progress, address concerns, and track improvements in blood pressure control and overall cardiovascular health.
By prioritizing regular check-ups, individuals with high blood pressure can stay informed about their health status, receive personalized care, and work towards achieving optimal blood pressure management. These routine medical visits provide opportunities for proactive interventions, timely adjustments to treatment plans, and ongoing support in promoting cardiovascular wellness and reducing the risk of complications associated with hypertension. Consistent engagement in regular check-ups fosters a collaborative approach to managing high blood pressure effectively and nurturing long-term health.

10. Understanding Blood Pressure Readings

Understanding blood pressure readings is essential for individuals with high blood pressure to monitor their cardiovascular health, assess the effectiveness of treatment, and make informed decisions about managing hypertension. Blood pressure readings consist of two numbers - systolic pressure (the top number) and diastolic pressure (the bottom number) - measured in millimeters of mercury (mm Hg). Here is a breakdown of interpreting blood pressure readings: Understanding Blood Pressure Readings:

1. Systolic Pressure:
 - The pressure within the arteries during a heartbeat and blood pumping is represented by the systolic pressure.
   - Normal systolic pressure is typically less than 120 mm Hg. Elevated systolic readings indicate increased pressure on artery walls during heart contractions.

2. Diastolic Pressure:
   - The diastolic pressure reflects the pressure in the arteries when the heart is at rest between beats.
   - A typical diastolic pressure is below 80 millibars. Elevated diastolic readings denote increased pressure on artery walls during relaxation phases of the heart.

3. Interpretation of Readings:
   - Blood pressure readings are categorized as follows:
     - **Normal:** Systolic less than 120 mm Hg and diastolic less than 80 mm Hg.
     - **Elevated:** Systolic between 120-129 mm Hg and diastolic less than 80 mm Hg.
     - Hypertension Stage 1: Systolic between 130-139 mm Hg or diastolic between 80-89 mm Hg.
     - Hypertension Stage 2: Systolic 140 mm Hg or higher or diastolic 90 mm Hg or higher.

4. Understanding Readings:
   - High blood pressure readings indicate increased pressure in the arteries, which can strain the heart,

damage blood vessels, and raise the risk of cardiovascular complications.
   - Consistently elevated blood pressure can lead to conditions such as heart disease, stroke, kidney damage, and vision problems.
5. Error Factors:
   - Factors such as stress, white coat hypertension (elevated readings in clinical settings), improper cuff size, recent caffeine consumption, and physical activity can affect blood pressure readings.
   - Monitoring blood pressure at home under optimal conditions can help reduce error factors and provide more accurate readings.
6. Personalized Targets:
   - Healthcare providers set personalized blood pressure targets based on individual health status, risk factors, and treatment goals.
   - Adjustments to treatment plans, lifestyle modifications, and medication regimens are made based on blood pressure readings and overall health assessments.
Understanding blood pressure readings empowers individuals to track their cardiovascular health, make proactive choices in managing high blood pressure, and collaborate with healthcare providers in optimizing treatment strategies. Regular monitoring and interpretation of blood pressure measurements support effective blood pressure control, reduce the risk of complications, and promote cardiovascular wellness. By staying informed about blood pressure readings, recognizing the significance of systolic and diastolic numbers, and

following personalized recommendations for managing hypertension, individuals can take charge of their cardiovascular health and work towards achieving optimal blood pressure levels.

Regular monitoring, interpretation, and communication of blood pressure readings with healthcare providers are integral components of managing high blood pressure effectively. By understanding the implications of blood pressure measurements, individuals can make informed decisions about lifestyle modifications, treatment options, and self-care practices to promote heart health, reduce the risk of complications, and improve overall quality of life. Consistent engagement in blood pressure monitoring, along with adherence to treatment recommendations and healthy lifestyle habits, supports long-term cardiovascular wellness and contributes to better outcomes for individuals with high blood pressure. Empowered by knowledge and proactive management strategies, individuals can navigate the complexities of hypertension with confidence, awareness, and a commitment to promoting heart-healthy behaviors.

11. Frequently Requested Information on Hypertension

High blood pressure, also known as hypertension, is a common medical condition characterized by elevated blood pressure levels in the arteries. It's a significant risk factor for various health complications, including heart disease, stroke, and kidney damage. As hypertension affects millions of people worldwide, it's natural for individuals to have questions about its causes, symptoms, treatment, and prevention. Here, we address some frequently asked questions about high blood pressure:

1. What is high blood pressure?
When there is a constant force of blood against the artery walls, high blood pressure results. This places increased strain on the heart and blood vessels, raising the risk of cardiovascular diseases.

2. What causes high blood pressure?
High blood pressure can have various causes, including genetics, lifestyle factors, and underlying health conditions such as obesity, diabetes, and kidney disease. Dietary factors such as excessive salt intake and insufficient potassium consumption can also contribute to hypertension.

3. What are the symptoms of high blood pressure?
In many cases, high blood pressure is asymptomatic, earning it the nickname "the silent killer." However, some individuals may experience symptoms such as headaches, dizziness, shortness of breath, and nosebleeds. It's essential to monitor blood pressure regularly, as untreated hypertension can lead to severe health complications.

4. How is high blood pressure diagnosed?

High blood pressure is typically diagnosed through blood pressure measurements taken with a sphygmomanometer. A diagnosis of hypertension is made when blood pressure consistently exceeds 130/80 mm Hg. Additional tests may be performed to assess for underlying health conditions contributing to high blood pressure.

5. What lifestyle changes can help manage high blood pressure?

Making changes to one's lifestyle is essential for controlling high blood pressure. These include adopting a heart-healthy diet rich in fruits, vegetables, whole grains, and lean proteins, limiting salt intake, maintaining a healthy weight, engaging in regular physical activity, limiting alcohol consumption, and quitting smoking.

6. What medications are used to treat high blood pressure?

In addition to lifestyle changes, healthcare providers may prescribe medications to lower blood pressure levels. These medications may include diuretics, ACE inhibitors, angiotensin II receptor blockers, beta-blockers, calcium channel blockers, and others. The choice of medication depends on individual factors such as age, overall health, and the presence of comorbid conditions.

7. Can high blood pressure be prevented?

While some risk factors for high blood pressure, such as genetics, cannot be changed, many lifestyle factors can be modified to reduce the risk. Adopting a healthy diet, maintaining a healthy

weight, exercising regularly, managing stress, limiting alcohol intake, and avoiding tobacco are essential strategies for preventing hypertension.
8. What are the complications of untreated high blood pressure? Unchecked high blood pressure can lead to severe health complications, including heart attack, stroke, heart failure, kidney disease, vision loss, and vascular dementia. It's crucial to manage hypertension effectively to reduce the risk of these complications and maintain overall health and well-being.
In conclusion, high blood pressure is a prevalent condition with significant implications for health and well-being. By understanding its causes, symptoms, diagnosis, treatment, and prevention strategies, individuals can take proactive steps to manage their blood pressure effectively and reduce the risk of associated complications. Regular monitoring, lifestyle modifications, and medical intervention when necessary are key components of a comprehensive approach to hypertension management.

12. Resources and Support for Individuals with High Blood Pressure

Individuals with high blood pressure can benefit from accessing various resources and support networks to help them manage their condition effectively. Here are some valuable resources and support options available for individuals with high blood pressure:

1. Healthcare Providers: Establishing a strong partnership with a trusted healthcare provider, such as a primary care physician or cardiologist, is essential for managing high blood pressure. Healthcare professionals can provide personalized guidance, medication management, and regular monitoring of blood pressure levels.

2. Educational Materials: Many reputable organizations, such as the American Heart Association (AHA) and the Centers for Disease Control and Prevention (CDC), offer educational materials and online resources about high blood pressure. These resources provide valuable information on risk factors, lifestyle modifications, treatment options, and prevention strategies.

3. Online Support Groups: Joining online support groups and forums dedicated to hypertension can provide individuals with a sense of community and connection. These platforms allow individuals to share experiences, exchange tips and advice, and offer support to one another in managing high blood pressure.

4. Mobile Apps: Several mobile applications are available specifically designed to help individuals track their blood pressure, monitor medication adherence, record lifestyle habits, and set health goals. These apps can serve as valuable tools for self-management and empowerment.

5. Community Wellness Programs: Many communities offer wellness programs and initiatives focused on

promoting heart health and preventing chronic diseases like hypertension. These programs may include fitness classes, nutrition workshops, stress management seminars, and blood pressure screenings.

6. Nutrition Counseling: Seeking guidance from a registered dietitian or nutritionist can be beneficial for individuals looking to adopt a heart-healthy diet to manage high blood pressure.These experts may help with meal planning, offer tailored dietary advice, and support in adopting sustainable lifestyle modifications.

7. Exercise Programs: Regular physical activity is essential for managing high blood pressure and improving overall cardiovascular health. Participating in structured exercise programs, such as aerobics classes, walking groups, or swimming sessions, can help individuals stay active and maintain a healthy weight.

8. Medication Assistance Programs: For individuals facing financial barriers to accessing prescribed medications for high blood pressure, medication assistance programs offered by pharmaceutical companies or nonprofit organizations may provide financial assistance or discounts on medications.

By utilizing these resources and support options, individuals with high blood pressure can take proactive steps to manage their condition effectively, reduce their risk of complications, and improve their quality of life. It's essential to explore and utilize the available resources to empower oneself in the journey towards better heart health.

Conclusion

In conclusion, high blood pressure is a serious health condition that requires proactive management and lifestyle modifications to reduce the risk of complications and improve overall health outcomes. By understanding the causes, symptoms, and risk factors associated with hypertension, individuals can take proactive steps to monitor their blood pressure, adopt a heart-healthy lifestyle, and seek appropriate medical care when necessary.

It's essential to recognize the importance of regular blood pressure monitoring, adherence to prescribed medications, and implementation of lifestyle modifications such as a healthy diet, regular exercise, stress management, and avoiding tobacco and excessive alcohol consumption. These lifestyle changes can significantly reduce blood pressure levels and lower the risk of heart disease, stroke, and other complications associated with hypertension.

Furthermore, seeking support from healthcare professionals, joining online support groups, accessing educational resources, and participating in community wellness programs can provide valuable support and encouragement on the journey to better heart health.

By taking proactive steps to manage high blood pressure, individuals can empower themselves to lead healthier, more fulfilling lives. Remember, small changes can make a big difference in managing blood pressure and reducing the risk of cardiovascular events. Together, let's prioritize heart health and strive towards a future where hypertension is effectively managed and its associated complications are minimized.

This table of contents provides a structured overview of key topics related to high blood pressure, covering essential information ranging from causes and symptoms to treatment options and prevention strategies. Feel free to customize and expand upon this outline further based on your specific requirements and the depth of information you wish to include.

www.ingramcontent.com/pod-product-compliance
Lightning Source LLC
Chambersburg PA
CBHW051856250726
48659CB00006B/2244